Irritable Syndrome

Roger Jones

Wolfson Professor of General Practice
Guy's, King's and St Thomas' School of Medicine
London UK

MARTIN DUNITZ

The views expressed in this publication are those of the author and not necessarily those of Martin Dunitz Ltd.

© 2001 Martin Dunitz Ltd, a member of the Taylor & Francis group

First published in the United Kingdom in 2001 by
Martin Dunitz Ltd
The Livery House
7–9 Pratt Street
London NW1 0AE

Tel: +44 (0)20 7482 2202
Fax: +44 (0)20 7267 0159
E-mail: info.dunitz@tandf.co.uk
Website: http://www.dunitz.co.uk

A CIP catalogue record for this book is available from the British Library.

ISBN 1-85317-985-X

Composition by Scribe Design, Gillingham, Kent
Printed and bound in Italy by Printer Trento S.r.l.

Contents

Contents

Introduction

Irritable bowel syndrome (IBS) has emerged from the relative obscurity of the 1960s and 70s, when it was a diagnosis of exclusion and often of last resort, to become a condition widely recognized as the cause of considerable morbidity, reduction in quality of life and costs to patients and health services. It is opportune to review the current state of knowledge of IBS at a time when our understanding of the causes of the condition has expanded considerably and new opportunities for management of the condition are becoming available.

Irritable bowel syndrome has enjoyed a chequered medical history, and some of the twists and turns of the story of functional bowel disorders are outlined in the first chapter, which concludes by bringing us up to date with current concepts of the definition of IBS and the criteria used for making a positive diagnosis. The ubiquity of IBS in the general population and in primary and secondary healthcare is emphasized in the second chapter, which also includes new data examining the interplay between the various symptom clusters that comprise the functional gastrointestinal (GI) disorders. Our understanding of the complex mechanisms likely to be involved in IBS is reviewed in the third chapter, in which gastrointestinal infection as a precursor to IBS is emphasized and the importance of adverse childhood life events and physical and sexual abuse is discussed. Subsequent chapters focus on the clinical presentations of IBS, noting the potentially confounding non-GI symptoms that may sometimes predominate over the abdominal problems, the principles of management of IBS and the importance of taking patients' concerns seriously and making a positive diagnosis. Separate chapters are devoted to drug and non-drug therapies and the evidence for their efficacy and their place in management. Finally, we look ahead to some of the clinical, research and educational challenges that we face in ensuring that patients with this difficult problem receive optimal therapy.

It is my hope that this pocketbook will act as a ready source of reference to both generalists and specialists interested in treating patients with IBS and also will widen the reader's understanding of some of the principles underlying patients' experience of functional somatic disorders, their interaction with the psychosocial dimensions of health and the best ways in which they can be understood, managed and alleviated.

Irritable bowel syndrome: history and disease definition

Introduction

Irritable bowel syndrome (IBS) is one of the **functional gastrointestinal disorders,** a term which covers a range of symptom complexes affecting the GI tract, and for which no organic cause has been demonstrated without doubt. These disorders range from non-ulcer dyspepsia and other upper GI syndromes, to functional abdominal bloating, constipation, diarrhoea and IBS itself. The cardinal features of IBS, which distinguish it from the other functional bowel disorders are:

- abdominal pain
- abdominal bloating or distension
- disordered defecation

IBS in the 19th century

Although irritable bowel syndrome is now an accepted term in the medical lexicon, it was not always so. Two sources from the early 19th century indicate the recognition of non-organic disorders of the GI tract but attribute them to 'a spasmodic stricture of the sigmoid flexure of the colon'. Writing in the *Medical Transactions* of the Royal College of Physicians in 1820, Powell described 'occasional pain in the intestines..., with flatulence and a sense of suffocation'; in 1830 Howship published a monograph entitled 'Practical remarks on the discrimination and successful treatment of spasmodic stricture in the colon'. The concept of some kind of mucosal inflammation dominated thinking about these disorders in the 19th century. Cumming, writing in the *London Medical Gazette* in 1849, described 'a peculiar affection of the mucous membrane of the bowels'. Therapies recommended at the time included enemas containing turpentine, castor oil and gruel and the use of the 'mustard blister' and electrogalvanism.

These unusual concepts of what we now recognize as IBS were perpetuated in the writings of the great Oxford and Baltimore physician, Sir William Osler. In his *Principles and Practice of Medicine* (published in 1892) Osler described 'mucous colitis', although he added that the colonic epithelium was normal in these cases: tellingly, he wrote that many patients were hysterical, hypochondriac, self-centred neurasthenic women. Osler's description included 'a tenacious mucus, which may be slimy and gelatinous, like frog spawn, which was passed in strings, strips or as a continuous tubular cast of the colon'. Osler recognized that some of these patients were likely to be constipated while others would have diarrhoea. These observations represent acute clinical descriptions of the syndrome, and also of physical signs encountered much less frequently in the 20th century. The brilliant Guy's Hospital physician, Sir Arthur Hurst, also described mucous colitis in a publication in the *Lancet* in 1836, labelling it 'the unhappy colon'. He reported that patients often brought mucous casts to the clinic and passed up to 50 grams of 'intestinal sand' in a day. It is unclear why these well-documented events are so very rarely seen in contemporary Western medicine.

IBS in the 20th century

Through the 20th century the nomenclature for IBS changed, even if the underlying physical symptoms did not.

The term **mucous colitis** gave way in the 1920s to 'colonic spasm and irritable colon' and in 1962 Chaudhary and Truelove coined the term 'irritable colon syndrome'. The first use of the term **irritable bowel syndrome** is attributed to DeLor, who published a paper of the same name in the *American Journal of Gastroenterology* in 1967. DeLor characterized IBS by one or a combination of symptoms including abdominal pain, diarrhoea, constipation, dyschezia and passage of mucus in the stool.

IBS: The modern era

In the 1970s, research in Bristol, UK by Heaton's group led to the publication of the **Manning criteria** (Table 1), which were the first diagnostic criteria used to identify patients with IBS. These were derived from a comparison of the presenting symptoms in two groups of patients referred to the hospital outpatients department – those who turned out to have functional (i.e. non-organic) complaints and those who turned out to have an organic cause for their symptoms. The criteria distinguish the functional from the organic patients; the more of the Manning symptoms a patient has, the more likely is the diagnosis of IBS.

Four symptoms were significantly more common among patients with IBS:
- looser stools at onset of pain
- more frequent bowel movements at onset of pain
- pain eased after bowel movement
- visible (abdominal) distension.

Two further symptoms were more common among patients with IBS:
- passage of mucus
- feeling of incomplete evacuation.

Table 1 The Manning criteria for diagnosis of IBS. Modified from Manning AP et al. *BMJ* 1978;**2**:653–4.

The Manning criteria stood the test of time for 20 years, and indeed are still used as the basis for making a positive diagnosis of IBS in primary care. However in specialist gastroenterology and for the purposes of research they are being replaced gradually by more recently developed diagnostic criteria. More precise diagnostic criteria for IBS were proposed in October 1986, at the 13th International Congress of Gastroenterology, and were subsequently published by Grant Thompson and colleagues in 1989 (Table 2).

Continuous or recurrent symptoms of:
1. Abdominal pain, relieved with defecation, or associated with a change in frequency or consistency of stool; *and/or*
2. Disturbed defecation (two or more of):
   * altered stool frequency
   * altered stool form (hard or loose/watery)
   * altered stool passage (straining or urgency, feeling of incomplete evacuation)
   * passage of mucus
   usually with
3. Bloating or feeling of abdominal distension.

Table 2 Diagnostic criteria for IBS. Modified from Thompson WG et al. *Gastroenterol Int* 1989;**2**:92–5.

Most recently, the Rome criteria have been developed (Tables 3, 4 and 5). These are more complex, restrictive and difficult to apply in practice than the criteria elaborated by Manning and Thompson and at present are mostly used as the basis for inclusion or exclusion of patients entering therapeutic trials of IBS.

At least 3 months continuous or recurrent symptoms of:
1. abdominal pain or discomfort which is:
    • relieved with defecation
    • and/or associated with a change in frequency of stool
    • and/or associated with a change in consistency of stool
    and
2. two or more of the following, at least a quarter of occasions or days:
    • altered stool frequency
    • altered stool form (lumpy/hard or loose/watery)
    • altered stool passage (straining or urgency, feeling of incomplete evacuation).
    • passage of mucus
    • bloating or feeling of abdominal distension.

Table 3 Rome criteria for diagnosis of IBS. Modified from Thompson WG et al. *Gastroenterol Int* 192;**5**:75–91.

At least 12 weeks, which need not be consecutive in the preceding 12 months of abdominal discomform or pain that has two of three features:
• relieved with defecation *and/or*
• onset associated with a change in frequency of stool *and/or*
• onset associated with a change in form (appearance of stool).

Table 4 Rome II criteria for diagnosis of IBS. Modified from Thompson WG et al. *Gut* 1999;**45**(suppl 2);1143–7.

The following symptoms cumulatively support the diagnosis of IBS:
• abnormal stool frequency
• abnormal stool form (lumpy/hard or loose/watery stool)
• abnormal stool passage (straining, urgency, or feeling of incomplete evacuation)
• passage of mucus
• bloating or feeling of abdominal distension.

Table 5 Rome II criteria for diagnosis of IBS. Modified from Thompson WG et al. *Gut* 1999;**45**(suppl 2):1143–7.

Diagnostic criteria in practice

In everyday practice, these formal criteria are rarely used. In a recent survey of general practitioners, it was found that most were unfamiliar with the Manning criteria (let alone the Rome criteria). Nonetheless, most of them diagnosed IBS with reasonable confidence. Their main concerns were the exclusion of organic disease (and two-thirds of them believed that their patient shared this concern), but few tests were ordered and over 70% of general practitioners (GPs) surveyed were prepared to make the diagnosis on the initial visit. The GPs in this study estimated that they referred only about one in seven IBS patients to specialists, the majority because of patient dissatisfaction and about one-third because of an uncertain diagnosis. Almost all GPs employed drug therapy, but they believed that the most important component of treatment was explanation and reassurance.

The principle of making an early, positive diagnosis, without over-investigation and unnecessary referral, is central to the effective management of IBS, and is discussed in detail later in this pocketbook.

Further reading

Manning AP, Thompson WG, Heaton KW, Morris AF. Towards positive diagnosis of the irritable bowel. *BMJ* 1978;**2**:653–4.

Thompson WG, Dotevall G, Drossman DA et al. Irritable bowel syndrome: Guidelines for diagnosis. *Gastroenterol Int* 1989;**2**:92–5.

Thompson WG, Creed F, Drossman DA et al. Functional bowel disease and functional abdominal pain. *Gastroenterol Int* 1992;**5**:75–91.

Thompson WG, Longstreth GF, Drossman DA, Heaton KW, Irvine EJ, Muller-Lissner SA. Functional bowel disorders and functional abdominal pain. *Gut* 1999;**45**(suppl 2):1143–7.

Thompson WG, Heaton KW, Smyth GT, Smyth C. Irritable bowel syndrome: the view from general practice. *Eur J Gastroenterol Hepatol* 1997;**9(7)**:689–92.

Epidemiology

Introduction

Community-based surveys of individuals not seeking health care indicate that GI symptoms are very common in the general population. These surveys have been conducted in many countries, particularly those in which a patient registration system operates in primary care. Dyspepsia, reflux symptoms, rectal bleeding and IBS are all experienced by a substantial proportion of individuals, and between one-quarter and one-third of these people become patients and seek formal health care for their problems.

Similarly, GI disorders are a common reason for consultation in primary care.

In the UK around 10% of all consultations with GPs concern GI disorders, with about half relating to upper GI problems (mostly dyspepsia, reflux and vomiting) and half to lower bowel symptoms, including IBS.

Prevalence of symptoms

- The **prevalence** of a condition describes the number of people identifiable with that condition over a specified time period. Hence, the six-month period prevalence of a disorder is the percentage of the population under study reporting that disorder during the six-month period.

- The **incidence** of a condition is a description of the number of new cases of the condition identified over a defined period; hence the annual incidence of IBS is the percentage of the study population presenting new IBS symptoms over a one-year period.

Estimates of the population prevalence of IBS vary quite widely around the globe. In North America and western Europe community-based surveys suggest that IBS affects 12–22% of the general population, whilst figures from South-East Asia indicate a prevalence of less than 5% (Figure 1). A survey undertaken in 1985 in New Zealand revealed a population prevalence of 14%, and a study performed in France in 1986 recorded a prevalence of 19%.

There may be several reasons for these different estimates. Different diagnostic criteria may be used, different survey methods (questionnaires, interviews, etc.) may be employed and the **denominator**, that is the size of the

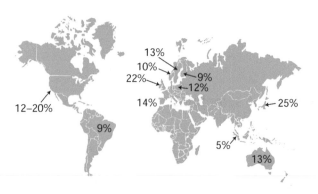

Figure 1 Population prevalence of IBS.

population under study, may be difficult to establish accurately. In countries with a widespread national registration system in primary care or general practice, the denominator is likely to be measurable with precision, but in other health-care settings this may be more difficult. Issues of literacy, access to patients and a number of other factors affecting the likely response to a survey instrument may also compromise the results.

The most recent large-scale survey, undertaken in the UK and involving over 4000 individuals who returned a validated postal questionnaire, indicated that the prevalence of IBS in the general population is in the region of 18%. The distribution of IBS in men and women is shown by age group in Figure 2.

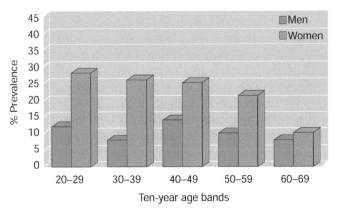

Figure 2 Prevalence of IBS.

Pattern of symptoms

When examining the way that the symptoms of IBS are distributed within and between patients and over time, three important messages emerge.

- First, patients can generally be classified into one of three IBS subtypes – diarrhoea-predominant, constipation-predominant or mixed;
- Second, the symptoms of IBS wax and wane over time, with a periodicity that varies between patients and often within patients;
- Third, for many patients a 'most bothersome' symptom can be identified and can act as an endpoint for successful treatment.

In a survey of patients in the south of England, Jones and Lydeard sent a validated postal questionnaire to over 2000 subjects randomly selected from a list of general practitioners; 22% of patients reported symptoms consistent with a diagnosis of IBS. The distribution of constipation and diarrhoea in the study population are shown in Figure 3; approximately equal proportions of patients reported either diarrhoea, constipation, alternating periods of diarrhoea or constipation, or neither symptom. As we will see later, the classification of IBS patients into one or other of these subtypes may be important in terms of targeting therapy. The old notion that all patients with IBS will respond to similar dietary manoeuvres, such as a high-fibre diet with lots of bran, has to be abandoned and replaced by a more

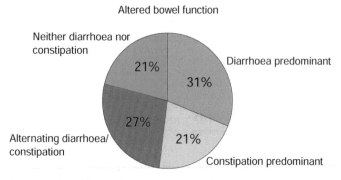

Figure 3 Altered bowel function in a population of patients with IBS. Modified from Jones RH, Lydeard S. *BMJ* 1992;**304**:87–90.

selective and sophisticated approach to diagnosis and choice of therapy.

The variation in the frequency, duration and severity of IBS symptoms and the pattern of individual episodes has only recently been studied in any depth, and the most helpful data have come from the use of an interactive telephone data entry system which patients use daily to record their symptoms. In a study from North America published by Hahn and colleagues, the majority of patients experienced at least one symptom of IBS on over half of the days during the study, but individual symptoms were reported on less than half of the days, indicating that different symptoms sometimes occurred sequentially rather than simultaneously. In other words IBS patients do not always experience all of their symptoms at the same time, and individual symptoms may occur or predominate on particular days. Overall, patients in this study reported the following:

- pain and discomfort on about one-third of days
- bloating on 28% of days
- altered stool form on 25% of days
- an altered pattern of defecation on 18% of days
- passage of mucus in the stool on 7% of days (Figure 4).

These findings are important in guiding clinicians' history-taking and also in terms of assessing patients' responses to therapy.

The concept of the 'most bothersome symptom' is an important one; although IBS is characterized by abdominal pain, bloating and changes in defecation, different patients may be more troubled by particular symptoms.

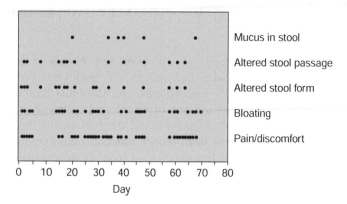

Figure 4 Symptom patterns in patients with IBS. Modified from GlaxoWellcome, data on file.

In a recent study Northcutt and colleagues asked patients participating in clinical trials the simple question "When your IBS is active, which of the following symptoms bothers you most?". Only one of a list of possible answers could be given, and the responses to this question are shown in Figure 5. It is clear that whilst over one-third of patients were most troubled by abdominal pain or discomfort, urgency of defecation, abdominal bloating and frequency of bowel movements were often more important for others;

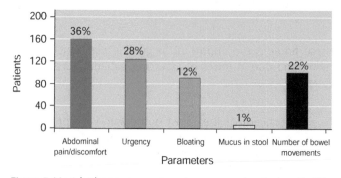

Figure 5 Most bothersome symptoms in a group of patients with IBS. Modified from Northcutt et al. *Gastroenterology* 1999;**116**:A1036.

the passage of mucus was rarely reported as the most bothersome symptom.

These data are also important in terms of clinical management; urgency of defecation may interfere so much with social activities that patients are more concerned to obtain relief of this symptom than of abdominal pain.

Natural history of IBS

The long-term course of IBS has not been very well studied in primary care or in the community, and most of our information relates to selected patients, often with more severe symptoms, seen in hospital outpatient departments. While many patients with IBS experience symptoms over a prolonged period, it seems likely that in other patients these symptoms may disappear or burn out after time. Agreus studied a Scandinavian population with functional bowel disorders; when following up patients' symptoms he found that there was movement between functional GI subgroups, so that some patients with non-ulcer dyspepsia developed symptoms of IBS whilst some patients with IBS reported dyspepsia as a more troublesome symptom at follow-up. On the other hand, whilst IBS tends to present in the first three decades of life, later presentations are not unknown, although new lower bowel symptoms in patients over the age of 45 years must be regarded with suspicion (see pages 34–5).

Further reading

Cabellero-Plascencia AM, Sofos-Kontoyannis S, Valenzuela-Barranco M, et al. Irritable bowel syndrome in patients with dyspepsia: a community based study in Southern Europe. *Eur J Gastroenterol Hepatol* 1999;**11**:517–22.

Ho KY, Kang JY, Seow A. Prevalence of gastrointestinal symptoms in a multiracial Asian population, with particular reference to reflux-type symptoms. *Am J Gastroenterol* 1998;**83**:1816–22.

Jones RH, Lydeard S. Irritable bowel syndrome in the general population. *BMJ* 1992;**304**:87–90.

Kennedy TM, Jones RH, Hungin AP et al. Irritable bowel syndrome, gastro-oesophageal reflux, and bronchial hyper-responsiveness in the general population. *Gut* 1998;**43**(6):770–4.

Hahn B, Watson M, Yan S et al. Irritable bowel syndrome symptom patterns. Frequency, duration and severity. *Dig Dis Sci* 1998;**43**:2715–8.

Northcutt AR, Harding JP, Kong S et al. Urgency as an endpoint in irritable bowel syndrome. *Gastroenterology* 1999;**116**:A1036.

Agreus L, Svardsudd K, Nyren O, Tibblin G. Irritable bowel syndrome and dyspepsia in the general population: overlap and lack of stability over time. *Gastroenterology* 1995;**109**(3):671–80.

Psychosocial factors

Introduction

This chapter describes the relationship of psychosocial factors to symptoms in IBS, the factors that are associated with patients' decisions to seek health care and the impact of IBS on individuals and on health-care systems, in terms of quality of life and the use of health-care resources.

Psychosocial factors in IBS

In early reports of functional lower bowel disorders an abnormal psychosocial profile, particularly anxiety, depression or 'neuroticism', was considered to be an integral part of the syndrome. This somewhat perjorative view persisted until relatively recently, when work from North America and Europe began to demonstrate that psychosocial dysfunction was not part of IBS *per se*, but was associated with health-care seeking behaviour. This discovery was made by conducting surveys of patients selected at random from the general population who were found to have symptoms compatible with a clinical diagnosis of IBS but had not consulted a physician. It was found that disorders such as anxiety and depression were more common in IBS sufferers seeking medical care than in those with IBS symptoms who did not seek professional advice. Furthermore there were few significant differences in the psychosocial characteristics of IBS patients seeking health care compared with other patients studied in ambulatory care settings, for example surgical outpatients.

These findings have important implications for understanding the pathogenesis of IBS, as they indicate that the symptoms do not develop as a result of psychosocial factors. They also impact on evaluation and management of the disorder, as patients seeking health care for IBS may well have significant psychopathology that might need treatment in its own right.

Health-care seeking in IBS

The community surveys described in the first chapter of this book showed that whilst IBS is extremely common in the general population, only about one-third of patients seek medical advice for their problems. It is important to understand the reasons for this and to be familiar with the concept of the iceberg of illness.

The pattern of consultation in IBS is shown diagrammatically in Figure 6. Most IBS sufferers do not seek medical advice. Within this group, as described earlier, symptoms are much more common in women than in men. About one-quarter of these patients enter primary care, once again with an approximately 2:1 female to male ratio (at

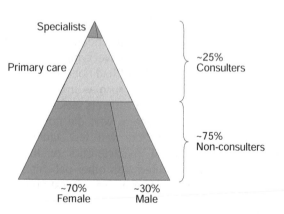

Figure 6 The pattern of consultation in IBS. Modified from Thompson WG, Drossman DA. *Gastroenterology* 1980;**79**:283–8.

least in Western societies). The female to male ratio is often reversed in non-Western countries, and this is thought to be an artefact of consultation behaviour rather than disease prevalence. The population seen by secondary and tertiary care specialists, indicated at the apex of the pyramid, represents a small and highly-selected population of IBS patients.

A number of factors play a role in the decision to seek medical advice:

- the presence of significant psychopathology
- the experience of recent threatening or adverse life events
- patients' fears that they may have cancer or a serious disease.

In an interview study of consulting and non-consulting IBS patients, both anxiety and depression were found to be much more common among the consulting group, who were also much more concerned that their symptoms represented a serious disease.

Despite the fact that only about one-quarter of IBS sufferers in the community consult physicians, IBS is the most frequently-made diagnosis among gastroenterologists and the fourth most common digestive disease diagnosis made by general practitioners. In primary care in the UK, IBS accounts for approximately one in eight consultations relating to the GI tract and in specialist practice it accounts for over one-quarter of gastroenterological diagnoses (Figure 7). Approaching 50% of gastroenterology practice involves the care of patients with functional GI disorders, and in some outpatient clinics up to 60% of follow-up appointments are related to functional bowel problems.

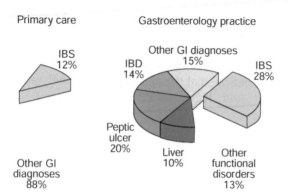

Figure 7 Diagnostic burden in the USA. Modified from Mitchell CM, Drossman DA. *Gastroenterology* 1987;**92**:1282–4.

Unsurprisingly patients with IBS are more likely to consult in both primary and secondary care and, to a lesser extent, in the emergency room. Recently published data from the both the USA and the UK indicate that IBS patients are significantly more likely than people without IBS to make use of primary and secondary care services.

Healthcare resources

In the USA IBS accounts for around three million physician visits each year and over two million prescriptions. In a community survey of over 4000 patients in the USA, Talley and colleagues found that one-year medical costs for a patient with IBS were significantly higher than those of other patients with GI symptoms or control patients without GI symptoms (Table 6). When Talley's group extrapolated their findings, based on costs collected in previous studies, they calculated that the annual cost of managing IBS in the USA was in the region of US$8 billion.

• Annual costs of health-care use	
• Patient with IBS	$742
• Patient with GI symptoms	$614
• Without GI symptoms	$429

Table 6 Financial burden of IBS – Direct costs in the USA. Modified from Talley NJ et al. *Gastroenterology* 1995;**109**:1736–41.

Similar work has been carried out in the UK, and recently Wells and colleagues estimated the annual expenditure on IBS in the UK to be in the region of £46 million (Table 7).

Estimate of annual expenditure	£45.6m
Based on the following costs:	
• GP consultations	£13.1m
• Prescribed medications	£12.5m
• Hospital outpatient visits	£16.6m
• Inpatient admissions	£ 3.4m

Table 7 Financial burden of IBS – Direct costs in the UK. Modified from Wells NEJ et al. *Aliment Pharamcol Ther* 1997;**11**:1019–30.

In addition to these direct costs to health services, which include the costs of consultations with physicians, diagnostic tests, prescriptions and hospitalizations, indirect costs related to IBS are also sustained by individuals and society. Hahn's work in the USA and the UK has indicated that IBS patients lose a significant proportion of working days and also experience a considerable number of days during which they are working at less than full productivity (Table 8). The same investigators reported significant excess of career problems (for example, job loss, refusal of promotion and the need to change jobs) in patients with IBS compared with non-IBS individuals.

Effect on work of IBS*	USA	UK
% sufferers who missed days	30.0	27.0
average number of days	1.7	1.8
% sufferers with reduced days	46.0	39.0
average number of days	3.0	2.5
*over previous 4 weeks.		

Table 8 Indirect costs of IBS in the UK and USA. Modified from Hahn BA et al. *Digestion* 1999;**60**:77–8.

Impact on quality of life

The importance of measuring aspects of patients' lives beyond simplistic measures of symptom severity and frequency is now widely recognized. Illness may impact on patients in many ways, including:

- physical functioning (sleep, sexual activity)
- mental health
- social interaction (work and leisure)
- general wellbeing and vitality.

A number of standard measuring instruments are available to assess quality of life, such as short form 36 (SF36), which is widely used to describe the impact of illness on patients. When SF36 is used to measure quality of life in patients with a variety of disorders, it is clear that IBS has a negative impact on quality of life that is comparable with the impact of clinical depression and more severe than that of type 2 diabetes (Figure 8). In the search for more sensitive measures of the impact of IBS on quality of life, other instruments have been devised, including the IBS QOL score; when IBS patients were compared with a theoretical normal value from non-IBS patients, Hahn demonstrated a significant reduction in quality of life across a number of dimensions (Figure 9).

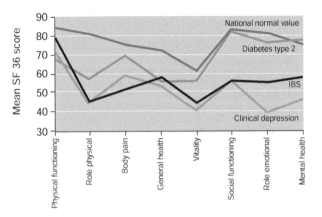

Figure 8 Quality of life compared with other diseases. Modified from Wells NEJ et al. *Aliment Pharmacol Ther* 1997;**11**:1019–30.

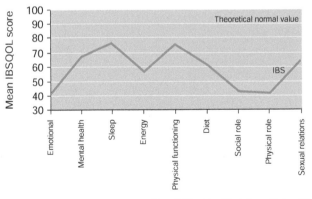

Figure 9 Negative impact on quality of life. Modified from Hahn BA, Kirchdoerfer LJ, Fullerton S, Mayer E. *Aliment Pharmacol Ther* 1997;**11**:547–52.

An awareness of the impact of IBS on patients' wellbeing in these various dimensions also has clear messages for clinical management, both in terms of evaluating patients at presentation and in assessing their response to therapy.

Further reading

Thompson WG, Drossman DA. Functional bowel disorders in apparently healthy people. *Gastroenterology* 1980;**79**:283–8.

Mitchell CM, Drossman DA. Survey of the AGA membership relating to patients with functional gastrointestinal disorders. *Gastroenterology* 1987;**92**:1282–4.

Kettell J, Jones RH, Lydeard S. Reasons for consultation in irritable bowel syndrome: symptoms and patient characteristics. *Br J Gen Pract* 1992,**42**:459–61.

Talley NJ, Gabriel SE, Harmsen WS, Zinsmeister AR, Evans RW. Medical costs in community subjects with irritable bowel syndrome. *Gastroenterology* 1995;**109**:1736–41.

Wells NEJ, Hahn BA, Whorwell PJ. Clinical economics review: irritable bowel syndrome. *Aliment Pharmacol Ther* 1997;**11**:1019–30.

Francis CY, Morris J, Whorwell PJ. The irritable bowel severity scoring system: a simple method of monitoring irritable bowel syndrome and its progress. *Aliment Pharmacol Ther* 1997;**11**:395–402.

Hahn BA, Yan S, Strassels S. Impact of irritable bowel syndrome on quality of life and resource use in the United States and United Kingdom. *Digestion* 1999;**60**:77–8.

Causes

Introduction

No single factor or abnormality capable of explaining all of the symptoms of IBS has been discovered, and probably none ever will be. Most recent research has pointed towards the need to think of an integrated model of the causes of IBS; in this model many factors, which are often studied in isolation, interact to produce the characteristics of the syndrome. There are few disease analogies with IBS, although the term 'the asthma of the gut', has been applied to IBS to emphasize some similarities between the two conditions. Both are common and intermittent conditions, although IBS is associated with a range of non-GI symptoms, whereas asthma is not.

Original theories about the causation of IBS began with colonic spasm and examination of intestinal motility dominated research for many years. The sensitivity of the GI tract was the next subject for research, followed by the way in which the enteric nervous system processes information arising in the gut, particularly painful and unpleasant stimuli. Most recently the importance of the entire brain–gut axis has been emphasized, as evidence has emerged from sophisticated research techniques that changes in the central processing of information arising in the gut may be important in IBS patients.

Motility

Intestinal spasm was initially thought to be the cause of pain in IBS, as a result of hypermotility in the affected part of the gut. Certainly the concept of a cramping pain or 'intestinal colic' provided not only a possible causative model, but also one which could be readily explained to patients. Unfortunately, the physiological abnormalities found in IBS patients are not consistent with a pure motility disorder; whilst patients with diarrhoea-predominant IBS may indeed have GI hypermotility, many IBS patients have normal or delayed intestinal transit, often accompanied by abnormalities of gastric emptying. Further, there is often within-patient variation in GI hypermotility, so that stool form as well as frequency varies over time.

Visceral causes

As research progressed and our understanding of IBS developed, attention shifted from abnormalities of motor function to concentrate on the sensitivity of the GI tract to unpleasant stimuli. A range of experiments were undertaken to show, for example, that the GI tract in people with IBS is more sensitive to balloon distension than that in normal individuals and that some IBS patients seem to have lower pain thresholds than controls (Figure 10). However once again, these abnormalities were unevenly distributed within and between IBS patients, and they did not explain many of the other abnormalities encountered in IBS.

It was not until the early 1980s that research began to explore in more detail the role of the enteric nervous system (ENS) in IBS and the important relationships between the gut and the brain.

The enteric nervous system

The enteric nervous system (ENS) is a subdivision of the autonomic nervous system, which is responsible for controlling bodily functions at a subconscious level.

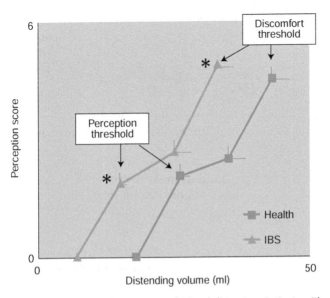

Figure 10 Dose-related perception of jejunal distension. Patients with IBS showed hypersensitivity to mechanoreceptor stimulation (*$P < 0.05$ vs controls). Reproduced with permission from Malagelada JR. *Aliment Pharmacol Ther* 1999;**13**(Suppl 2):57–64.

The ENS contains numerous reflex pathways that control contractions of the smooth muscle of the alimentary tract, intestinal secretions, water and electrolyte transport, mucosal blood flow and other functions. There are connections and interactions between the ENS and the sympathetic and parasympathetic systems, and also with sensory and motor nerves. Neurones from the ENS innervate:

- the GI mucosa
- the muscularis mucosa
- the submucosa
- the circular and longitudinal muscles of the GI tract
- the myenteric plexus.

Perhaps of most relevance to IBS, it seems that descending neural pathways from the brain are capable of modulating the activity of afferent visceral pathways which convey sensory information from the gut. This may represent one mechanism whereby activity in higher centres in the central nervous system can influence the way in which sensations arising in the gut are perceived by patients and also the way that the gut responds to stimulation.

The ENS contains almost as many neurotransmitters as the brain itself, and these include, among many others:

- a number of 5–hydroxytryptamine (5HT) derivatives
- acetylcholine
- opioids
- somatostatin
- substance P
- vasoactive intestinal polypeptide.

Some neurones appear to contain several, often as many as five, different possible neurotransmitters. Although the pathological role of neurotransmitter abnormalities within ENS has not been clearly defined, research interest has focused on agents capable of modifying neurotransmission within the system. The $5HT_3$ and $5HT_4$ transmitters, which seem to be involved in abnormalities of the gut such as changes in peristaltic response, colonic motility and fluid secretion, have been the subject of considerable study. These studies have led to the development of promising therapeutic agents for IBS, which appear to have their action either as agonists or antagonists of the $5HT_3$ and $5HT_4$ receptors in the ENS.

Brain–gut interaction

Whilst abnormalities in motility, sensitivity and signalling in the GI tract and ENS may well account for some of the symptoms experienced by patients with IBS, the intensity of discomfort experienced and the degree of derangement of intestinal function may well be mediated by the neuronal connections between the gut and the brain (Figure 11).

Brain–gut interaction can take place in a number of ways, all of which potentially overlap and interact. At the most physical level it is possible that brain efferent neural pathways, described above, modulate signals resulting from gut activity and influence gut function. At a higher level of processing, there is increasing evidence that information may be processed differently by patients with IBS compared with normal people. For example, using PET (positon emission tomography) scanning, it appears that IBS patients' thalamic activity is different from that in non-IBS individuals. There is also evidence of hypervigilance in

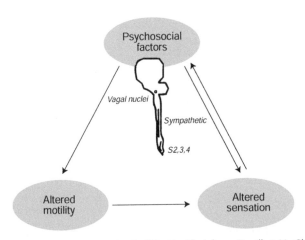

Figure 11 Brain–gut interaction in IBS. Modified from Camilleri M, Choi M.G. *Aliment Pharmacol Ther* 1997;**11**:3–15.

IBS patients; in experiments involving the threat of unpleasant stimuli, there is evidence of enhanced frontal lobe activity in IBS patients compared with controls.

All of these physical neurochemical interactions are complicated by the much more subtle interplay between psychological state, the social milieu and the experience of discomfort. Health-care seeking behaviour and illness onset may be precipitated by adverse life events, and many symptoms are likely to be more severe and to be presented to doctors when there is a background of depression or anxiety (Figure 12). In an analogy to the hypervigilant state demonstrated by PET scanning, IBS patients may 'fear the worst', leading to the generation of automatic negative thinking about bowel symptoms, and associated therapeutic nihilism. Indeed, the negative connotations placed by IBS sufferers on visceral sensations offer one opportunity for the use of cognitive behavioural therapy in IBS.

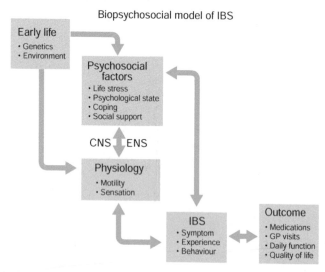

Figure 12 Biopsychosocial model of IBS. Drossman DA. An integrated approach to the irritable bowel syndrome. *Aliment Pharmacol Ther* 1999;**13**(suppl 2):3–14.

Postinfective IBS

This is important, as it has become clear that as many as one-third of patients with IBS appear to have suffered some kind of acute GI infective episode in the month before their symptoms developed. This may be a viral gastroenteritis or an infection with an organism such as *Giardia* or *Amoeba*. In any event, the symptoms of gastroenteritis subside but bloating, abdominal pain and frequently a diarrhoea-predominant IBS emerge. Carefully analysed electron microscope histological samples from these patients frequently reveal changes reminiscent of those seen in inflammatory bowel disease and, indeed, there are case reports of dramatic response to immuno-suppressant therapy. There is, of course, a further analogy here with bronchial hyperreactivity developing after an acute respiratory infection. Identifying postinfective IBS may be important, because there is obvious scope for therapeutic intervention, although no measures have been shown to be effective in randomized trials thus far.

Sexual and physical abuse

Although the precise links between the development of IBS and a history of childhood or adult sexual or physical abuse are difficult to define, there is evidence, mostly from the USA, that IBS patients are more likely to have experienced abuse and that this association exists independently of health-care seeking behaviour for other conditions. Although still somewhat controversial, it may be important to enquire sympathetically about this sensitive area when evaluating patients with difficult IBS symptoms.

Further reading

Farthing MJG. Irritable bowel, irritable body or irritable brain? *BMJ* 1995;**310**:171–5.

Drossman DA. An integrated approach to the irritable bowel syndrome. *Aliment Pharmacol Ther* 1993;**13**(suppl 2):3–14.

Gershon MD. Roles played by 5–hydroxytryptamine in the physiology of the bowel. *Aliment Pharmacol Ther* 1999;**13**(suppl 2):15–30.

Collins S, Barbara G, Vallance B. The putative role of inflammation in functional bowel disorders. In: Goebell H, Holtmann G, Tolley N (eds). *Functional dyspepsia and the irritable bowel syndrome*. Dordrecht: Kluwer; 1998: 135–9.

Garcia Rodriguez LA, Ruigomez A. Increased risk of irritable bowel syndrome after bacterial gastroenteritis: cohort study. *BMJ* 1999;**318**:565–6.

Ratcliffe J, Creed F. Sexual abuse and irritable bowel syndrome: the debate goes on. In: Goebell H, Holtmann G, Tolley N (eds). *Functional dyspepsia and the irritable bowel syndrome*. Dordrecht: Kluwer; 1998: 198–204.

Clinical presentations

Introduction

Although the diagnostic criteria – Manning, Thompson, Rome, etc. – delineate the symptom complex in patients with 'typical' IBS, the presentation, evaluation and diagnosis of patients with this syndrome is not always straightforward:

- First, psychosocial and physical factors interact, and may confuse the picture.
- Second, IBS may mimic other conditions, such as biliary tract disease and pelvic disorders, because of atypical location of pain.
- Third, IBS is often accompanied by other extra-GI symptoms, such as low back pain, migraine, urinary tract symptoms, and asthma/bronchial hyperreactivity, all of which are encountered more frequently than expected in patients with IBS.

Typical presentations

In Western medicine, most patients presenting in primary care with IBS are women in their 20s and 30s. The commonest presenting symptom is pain, followed by abdominal distension and an abnormality of bowel habit. Passage of rectal mucus is often not volunteered and is by no means a constant feature (Table 9).

- Abdominal pain
- Abdominal distension
- Change in bowel habit
- Pain eased by defecation
- Looser or more frequent stools at the onset of pain
- Passage of mucus *per rectum*

Table 9 Typical presenting features of IBS

The diagnosis of IBS may evolve over time. Patients frequently present in general practice and primary care with a partially developed syndrome (this is true for many other conditions, as well as IBS) so that there may be a number of consultations with a GP before the diagnosis becomes absolutely clear. For example, a patient may report one or two episodes of abdominal pain without much in the way of diarrhoea or constipation and it may only be with the occurrence of a more typical presentation, such as abdominal bloating, that the diagnosis can be made.

IBS presents less commonly in older patients, but with advancing age the possibility of an underlying organic problem must be borne in mind. The concept of alarm symptoms in evaluation of patients with GI disorders is important, and the alarm symptoms for lower bowel malignancy are listed in Table 10. Middle-aged or older patients presenting with these symptoms should be referred swiftly for specialist investigation, as appropriate.

IBS and psychopathology

As the association between seeking health care and psychopathology in IBS is well established newly-presenting IBS patients may have significant anxiety, depression or

- New symptoms over the age of 50 years
- Rectal bleeding
- Weight loss
- Feeling of incomplete evacuation
- Strong family history of colorectal cancer
- History of inflammatory bowel disease

Table 10 Alarm symptoms for lower bowel malignancy

other psychiatric dysfunction, as well as acute or ongoing social or domestic difficulties. In making an early diagnosis and deciding on appropriate therapy, it is important to make a thorough assessment of a patient's mental state as well as the extent of their GI symptoms.

Extra-GI symptoms in IBS

A number of studies have shown that both IBS subjects in the general population and IBS patients presenting in primary and secondary care are likely to report a range of associated symptoms that appear to have their origin outside the GI tract. Whorwell's group documented that IBS patients are more likely to complain of fatigue, back pain, fibromyalgia and migraine; Jones and Lydeard reported an excess of migraine and urinary tract symptoms (but not asthma) in their community-based study from the south of England; and most recently Kennedy and colleagues showed that asthma and bronchial hyperreactivity, migraine and urinary tract symptoms are more commonly reported in IBS patients than in non-IBS individuals (Table 11). In the same survey it was shown that IBS patients were more likely to have had a hysterectomy and a cholecystectomy than non-IBS patients (Table 12). IBS patients are also more likely to have functional dyspepsia and gastro-oesophageal reflux.

	IBS	Non-IBS
Asthma	24%	12%
Migraine	43%	26%
Urinary symptoms (women)	40%	21%

Table 11 Prevalence of extra-GI problems in IBS patients

	IBS	Non-IBS
Hysterectomy	18.0%	12.0%
Cholecystectomy	4.5%	2.4%

Table 12 Hysterectomy and cholecystectomy in IBS patients

The association between IBS and some of these symptoms, which appear to have their origin in smooth muscle dysfunction, is of considerable interest. For example IBS patients have been shown to have an abnormal bronchoconstrictor response to methacholine challenge compared with non-IBS controls. In addition, detrusor muscle function has been shown to be abnormal in over half of IBS patients compared with non-IBS controls. Whether these findings have real implications for further understanding the pathogenesis of IBS is uncertain but it is clear that the co-presentation of these potentially confusing symptoms can lead not only to misdiagnosis but also to inappropriate referral and, almost certainly, to inappropriate surgery.

Atypical presentations in IBS

These findings mean that physicians need to have a relatively high diagnostic index of suspicion for IBS in patients presenting with non-specific or unusual abdominal symptoms. For example, the location of pain in IBS may be atypical, so that confusion with biliary tract disease in patients with predominantly right upper quadrant pain is possible. Perhaps more difficult to diagnose are women whose pain is not cyclical but is located in the pelvis and iliac fossae, and for which a gynaecological, rather than GI, cause is thought to be likely. It is probable that many patients previously diagnosed as having 'chronic pelvic pain' or 'pelvic congestion' are, in reality, suffering from IBS.

The practical implication of these potentially confusing clinical presentations is that the diagnostic criteria put forward by Manning and Thompson need to be borne in mind when taking a history.

> Irrespective of the typical nature or site of the abdominal pain, a history of abdominal bloating and disordered defecation, possibly with the passage of mucus *per rectum* should be sought, and the possibility of a GI cause for these otherwise unexplained symptoms seriously considered.

Further reading

Kennedy TM, Jones RH, Hungin AP, O'Flanagan H, Kelly P. Irritable bowel syndrome, gastro-oesophageal reflux, and bronchial hyper-responsiveness in the general population. *Gut* 1998;**43**:770–4.

Maxton DG, Morris J, Whorwell PJ. More accurate diagnosis of irritable bowel syndrome by the use of 'non-colonic' symptomatology. *Gut* 1991;**32**:784–6.

Prior A, Wilson K, Whorwell PJ, Faragher EB. Irritable bowel syndrome in the gynaecological clinic. Survey of 798 new referrals. *Dig Dis Sci* 1989;**34**:1820–4.

Whorwell PJ, Lupton EW, Erduran D, Wilson K. Bladder smooth muscle dysfunction in patients with irritable bowel syndrome. *Gut* 1986;**27**:1014–17.

Whorwell PJ, McCallum M, Creed FH, Roberts CT. Non-colonic features of irritable bowel syndrome. *Gut* 1986;**27**:37–40.

Management

Introduction

The principles of managing patients with IBS are based not only on an understanding of the epidemiology, natural history and pathophysiology of the condition, but also on an awareness of the reasons that patients with IBS decide to seek medical advice. As lower bowel symptoms in account for perhaps 5% of all consultations in general practice, GPs need to develop a management approach that ensures timely diagnosis of functional bowel disorders without over-investigation. At the same time, they must retain an appropriate level of diagnostic suspicion, so that more serious disease (inflammatory bowel disease and cancer) is not overlooked.

Clinical presentation

We have seen that the peak onset for IBS is in the late 20s age group and that more women than men are affected. Pain is likely to be the predominant symptom in many cases, necessarily accompanied by a change in bowel habit and generally by abdominal bloating, although the importance and severity of these symptoms in an individual patient may change over time. It is probably important, in terms of obtaining an accurate clinical picture, to try to determine which is the **predominant** symptom for an individual patient and, as far as possible, to target treatment to that symptom.

We know that most general practitioners still do not use the Manning criteria, let alone the Rome criteria, yet they are reasonably accurate in making diagnoses in patients with functional bowel disorders. This means that both the sensitivity and specificity of the clinical diagnosis of IBS in general practice are relatively low, so that we are bound to encounter false negatives and false positives.

> A management strategy for primary care needs to be developed to minimize over-diagnosing IBS when it is not present (false positives) and not diagnosing the condition when it is present (false negatives).

It may be, for example, that 'missed' cases of inflammatory bowel disease have been diagnosed as IBS in the past, in patients in whom pain and bloating predominated and rectal bleeding and severe diarrhoea were absent. Conversely some patients without IBS but with relatively trivial digestive symptoms may have been inappropriately labelled as having the condition, leading to unnecessary anxiety and investigation (Table 13).

- Inflammatory bowel disease
- Malabsorption/dietary factors
- Infection
- Neoplasia
- Psychopathology
- Biliary tract disease
- Pelvic disease

Table 13 Differential diagnosis in IBS

Health beliefs and psychosocial examination

The importance of addressing patients' concerns and attempting to tease out their reasons for seeking medical advice cannot be over-emphasized. IBS is no different from any other condition in this respect; not listening to patients is a potent cause of misdiagnosis and inappropriate management, with adverse consequences for all concerned.

We have seen in previous chapters how physical, social and psychological factors interact in IBS, and an exploration of all three aspects needs to be undertaken. Depending on the physician's knowledge of the patient, an exploration of past as well as present social, domestic and psychological issues may be required (Table 14).

- Listen to patients' concerns
- Take health beliefs seriously
- Explanation, then reassurance
- Honest account of likely course of disease
- Minimal initial investigation
- Realistic expectations
- Provide continuity of care

Table 14 Principles of management of IBS

Two characteristics of diagnosis and management in primary care are the need to live with uncertainty and the use of time as a diagnostic (and sometimes therapeutic) tool. This is true in IBS, where time can be used to allow the symptom complex to evolve and clarify and to resolve the initial uncertainty about the diagnosis, which may take a number of consultations. In parallel, an exploration of the psychosocial milieu can sometimes be deferred to subsequent consultations when examination of sensitive issues, perhaps including sexual or physical abuse, can be undertaken in a more relaxed atmosphere.

Evaluation and investigation

> Standard advice to general practitioners is to make a positive diagnosis of IBS as soon as possible.

In an ideal world, we would all do this on the basis of a patient's presenting symptoms, an appropriate discussion of psychosocial issues and a limited physical examination. In reality, as described above, certain patients may present a rather more diffuse set of symptoms and the diagnosis may emerge over time. Nonetheless it is important, whenever possible, to make a diagnosis and communicate it to the patient as quickly as possible.

Making the diagnosis depends on a sympathetically taken history, a careful physical examination and the minimum of investigations. The importance of history taking and listening has already been discussed. A physical examination should **always** be performed including, if appropriate, a digital rectal examination to assure the patient that the symptoms are being taken seriously and to be absolutely certain that no major organic lesion is overlooked, particularly in older patients. Investigations should be kept to a minimum, although their role in the initial work-up of IBS varies from country to country. In the UK, unless patients have any of the alarm symptoms mentioned earlier (particularly new symptoms in middle age and beyond) it is appropriate to check a full blood count, ESR and perhaps a guaiac stool test for occult GI blood loss. In younger patients, investigations are not recommended at this early stage (Table 15).

In other western European countries the work-up in primary care may include tests for lactose intolerance, coeliac disease and pancreatic exocrine insufficiency, accompanied by endoscopy and radiology. These differences in approach reflect the characteristics of the health-

- FBC + ESR/CRP
- Sigmoidoscopy
- Stool for blood/infection
- Imaging
- Lactose intolerance?
- Malabsorption?

FBC, full blood count; ESR, erythrocyte sedimentation rate;
CRP, C-reactive protein.

Table 15 IBS: Further investigations to consider

care system in which the patients seek medical attention
and the nature and level of specialization of primary care
physicians.

With an understanding of the theoretical background of
IBS and an awareness of the Manning and Rome criteria,
most GPs should be able to make an accurate clinical
diagnosis of IBS after the first two or three consultations.
The next crucial step in management is accurate communication to the patient. We need to choose words that
patients can understand and to be realistic about IBS,
communicating the fact that it is not a life-threatening
illness but also being open about the fact that it is likely
to recur from time to time and can be troublesome. We
need to back this up with a reassurance that medical advice
can be sought when necessary and that a number of
measures are available to treat or minimize the symptoms.
These are discussed in the final chapters of this book on
drug and non-drug therapies.

Investigation and referral

Patients in whom we have made a confident diagnosis of
IBS may fail to obtain relief from lifestyle advice, dietary
advice, pharmacological treatment and non-drug therapies,

and some of these will, as we all know, become chronic attenders. The reason for the development of an 'illness career' by some IBS patients is not well understood, but may relate to poor communication about the nature of the diagnosis and its prognosis at an early stage. However, there are undoubtedly some patients whose symptoms present a real challenge and in whom further investigation and specialist referral need to be considered.

> In primary care, concerns about the presence of an organic cause for refractory bowel symptoms dominate diagnostic thinking.

Even when screening blood tests are normal, concern may still exist about the possibility that inflammatory or neoplastic disease is responsible for the patient's symptoms. In these cases, and where direct access to endoscopy and radiology is available, it is entirely appropriate for the GP to arrange further investigations to rule out these conditions, explaining carefully to the patient the reason for the tests. However, reassurance can be addictive, and patient pressure for further investigations should be resisted if at all possible.

The place of specialist referral is controversial, and the need for it depends to a large extent on an individual general practitioner's willingness to tolerate uncertainty and diagnostic disappointment. The danger, of course, is that patients enter the hospital outpatient system where they again become chronic attenders who are unnecessarily over-investigated by a succession of junior hospital staff, and who develop a dependence on the next test and the next trial of therapy. There is a strong argument that patients with IBS referred by GPs should be seen by a senior gastroenterologist at the first encounter, so that this situation does not develop. Gastroenterology clinics in which physicians work closely with psychologists or psychiatrists have much to offer, and it is likely that patients will benefit from a 'dual diagnostic' approach of this kind.

Finally IBS patients are frequently mis-referred to specialties other than gastroenterology, most notably general surgery and gynaecology. IBS patients seem to have an excess of cholecystectomies and hysterectomies, and this may well be the result of mis-attribution of symptoms to an organic origin, for which surgery seems appropriate. This is a difficult situation to change, but it depends in part on specialists being equally aware of the range of symptoms that can develop in IBS and thinking broadly about possible diagnoses outside the system in which they specialize.

Further reading

Farthing MJG. Irritable bowel, irritable body or irritable brain? *BMJ* 1995;**310**:171–5.

Drossman DA. An integrated approach to the irritable bowel syndrome. *Aliment Pharmacol Ther* 1993;**13**(Suppl 2):3–14.

Drug therapy

Introduction

Most patients with IBS are likely to receive some form of drug treatment to deal with their most troublesome symptoms. A range of drugs is available for treatment of IBS, although the clinical trial evidence for the efficacy of some of them is relatively thin. In the initial work-up of IBS patients, information about the time relationships of symptoms to external factors, including meals and specific foods, will have been discussed. Advice about appropriate dietary patterns and mealtimes will have been given; more detailed advice on dietary measures in IBS is provided in the next chapter.

> The choice of drug treatment in IBS is related to an assessment of an individual patient's most troublesome symptoms.

Symptoms are likely to include one or more of:

> - abdominal pain
> - abdominal bloating
> - constipation
> - diarrhoea

As we have seen, between one-third and one-half of IBS patients tend to have a mixed picture, with alternating constipation and diarrhoea; the remainder are split roughly equally between diarrhoea-predominant and constipation-predominant IBS.

Clinical trials in IBS

The difficulty facing the practising physician is that no single drug has been shown to be universally effective in IBS, and the wide range of drugs currently used in various countries reflects the unpredictable response of patients to drug therapy.

There have been many problems in establishing the efficacy of drugs used to treat IBS. One is that we have a relatively poor understanding of the syndrome, so that the design of randomized trials and the definition of inclusion and exclusion criteria has often been very difficult. The new Rome criteria may help in this regard, and most current therapeutic trials now focus either on abdominal pain or the patient's most predominant symptom as an outcome measure or on a global assessment of efficacy. Second, and perhaps most difficult to deal with, is the very high **placebo response** in IBS patients. In most placebo-controlled trials 30–50% of patients respond to the inactive drug, and so the opportunity for therapeutic gain in these trials is reduced. Many earlier therapeutic trials employed agents with a mode of action that was poorly understood; these agents are now recognized as being inappropriate on the basis of our current understanding of the pathogenesis of IBS.

Two recent meta-analyses of the use of antispasmodic agents in IBS came to different conclusions, so that the evidence for their routine use in IBS remains weak. Nonetheless, antispasmodics such as mebeverine and alverine are widely used and alverine is frequently purchased by patients as an over-the-counter medication.

IBS drugs

A number of drugs that are specifically licensed for the treatment of IBS are available for primary care physicians, although different selections of drugs are available in different countries. Overall, most of the drugs commonly prescribed in primary care are anticholinergic compounds, designed to reduce smooth muscle spasm. In the UK these agents include:

- propantheline
- hyoscine
- dicyclomine
- alverine
- mebeverine

In Australia a mixture of hyoscine, atropine and scopolamine is available. In Canada, hyoscyamine and in France prifinium are used. A further selection of drugs without anticholinergic properties is also used to treat IBS. For example, peppermint oil has a carminative action, but as well as possibly improving lower bowel symptoms it may aggravate gastro-oesophageal reflux, which is known to occur more frequently in IBS patients. Trimebutane is an opiate antagonist, with possible analgesic actions and an effect on GI spasm. Finally, in Canada the calcium channel blocker pinaverium is also used to treat IBS symptoms.

At present, it is difficult to provide clear advice about the use of these drugs, designed for the 'global' treatment of IBS. Whilst randomized controlled evidence for their efficacy is uncertain, there is no doubt that some patients benefit from them, particularly when given in higher dosage.

In practice, the primary care physician requires a therapeutic agent with predictable efficacy to back up advice about pathogenesis and prognosis in IBS; none of the currently used agents described above are sufficiently effective to meet this requirement.

Fortunately, as our understanding of the complex neuropharmalogical characteristics of the enteric nervous system improves, new therapeutic opportunities are revealed. Particular interest has focused in recent years on a number of transmitters and receptors, particularly $5HT_3$ and $5HT_4$. Drugs with antagonist and agonist effects on $5HT_3$ and $5HT_4$ receptors appear to have differential effects on bowel function, so that $5HT_3$ antagonists, for instance, appear to reduce symptoms of pain and diarrhoea in subjects with diarrhoea-predominant IBS. The $5HT_4$ partial agonist, tegaserod has been shown to have a therapeutic effect in patients with slow transit and constipation-predominant IBS, as illustrated in the accompanying figures, summarizing data from recent therapeutic trials. This is an area of intense research activity, and studies in progress are likely to yield further insights into the role of a range of neurotransmitters in the enteric nervous system and the therapeutic opportunities that this understanding provides.

Symptom-focused management

While there are reservations about drugs licensed for the overall treatment of IBS, there is no doubt that several groups of drugs have an important therapeutic role in the management and control of specific IBS-related symptoms. In patients with diarrhoea-predominant IBS, for example, antidiarrhoeal agents such as loperamide, diaphenoxylate and cholestyramine are all useful.

When constipation is predominant, besides dietary manipulation, the addition of unprocessed bran to meals taken two or three times a day is often effective; bulking agents such as ispaghula husk and psyllium can also be given with good effect.

The pain of IBS often presents problems, particularly when antispasmodics are ineffective. There is some

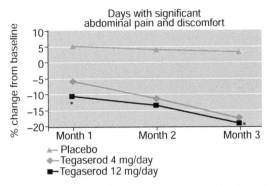

Figure 13 Effect of tegaserod on APD. *P<0.05 vs. placebo. Modified from Lefkowitz M et al. *Am J Gastroenterol* 1999;**94**:2676.

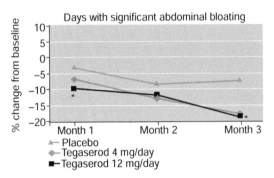

Figure 14 Effect of tegaserod on abdominal bloating. *P<0.05 vs. placebo. Modified from Krumholz S et al. *Gut* 1999;**45**:(Suppl5).

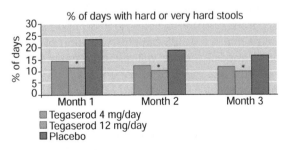

Figure 15 Effect of tegaserod on bowel function (stool consistency). *P<0.05 vs. placebo. Modified from Lefkowitz et al. *Am J Gastroenterol* 1999;**94**:2676.

evidence that dicyclomine is effective, although when diarrhoea coexists with pain, opiate-related analgesics such as codeine phosphate and dextropropoxyphene may be considered.

Antidepressant medication

The role of antidepressant medication in IBS is controversial. There is no doubt that when clinical depression can be identified on the basis of a mental state examination, antidepressants should be given in full doses. There is some evidence that tricyclic antidepressants are more efficacious in this condition than the newer selective serotinin reuptake inhibitors, such as paroxetine and fluoxetine, but the trial evidence for the use of low-dose tricyclic antidepressants is scanty. There is, however, some recent evidence from functional PET (positron emission tomography) scanning of the brains of patients with IBS that low doses of both classes of antidepressants have a direct central effect on the processing of visceral sensations, which may be beneficial in IBS.

Over-the-counter drugs

Although the arrangements for obtaining prescribed and over-the-counter (OTC) drugs vary from country to country, it is important to realize that many IBS patients who do not seek formal medical advice will obtain information and drug treatment from community pharmacists.

Bulking agents, peppermint oil and antispasmodics are now widely sold in the UK, although little information is currently available about the impact that these newly available drugs have had on the natural history of IBS in non-consulting patients. Clearly community pharmacists have a potentially important role in providing advice and treatment but they also face the challenge of evaluating patients with potentially serious lower bowel symptoms who are choosing to seek advice from a pharmacy rather than a primary care physician.

Further reading

Jones RH, Holtmann G, Rodrigo L et al. Alosetron relieves pain and improves bowel function compared with mebeverine in female nonconstipated irritable bowel syndrome patients. *Aliment Pharmacol Ther* 1999;**13**:1419–27.

Camilleri M, Mayer EA, Drossman DA et al. Improvement in pain and bowel function in female irritable bowel patients with alosetron, a 5–HT3 receptor antagonist. *Aliment Pharmacol Ther* 1999;**13**:1149–59.

Chapman ND, Grillage MG, Maxumder R, Atkinson SN. A comparison of mebeverine with high-fibre dietary advice and mebeverine plus isphaghula in the treatment of irritable bowel syndrome: an open, prospectively randomised, parallel group study. *Br J Clin Prac* 1990;**44**:461–6.

Poynard T, Naveau S, Mory B, Chaput JC. Meta-analysis of smooth muscle relaxants in the treatment of irritable bowel syndrome. *Aliment Pharmacol Ther* 1994;**8**:499–510.

Scarpignato C, Pelosini I. Management of irritable bowel syndrome: novel approaches to the pharmacology of gut motility. *Can J Gastroenterol* 1999;**13**(Suppl A):50A–65A.

Scott LJ, Perry CM. Tegaserod. *Drugs* 1999;**53**:491–6; 497–8.

Non-drug therapy

Introduction

The treatment of IBS begins with the first consultation and it is likely that the doctor–patient interaction at this time and in subsequent early encounters will set the pattern of health-care seeking behaviour and management, to a large extent, for the future. The crucial importance of taking a patient-centred approach in individuals with functional bowel disorders has already been emphasized, and the dangers of omitting to do so have been underlined. Patients need to be taken seriously, to be listened to and treated with respect. Patients' expectations are ever-rising and, as a wide range of medical information becomes available from electronic sources, their level of knowledge is greater than ever. General practitioners and other primary care physicians must recognize that a traditional paternalistic relationship, where reassurance consists of little more than a pat on the back, will no longer be regarded as adequate by most patients.

A range of non-drug therapies contributes to the management of IBS. These include:

- dietary advice
- exclusion diets where appropriate
- informal patient-centred consultations
- counselling
- formal psychotherapy (including cognitive behavioural therapy)
- hypnosis
- some complementary therapies.

Informal treatment

The GP and psychoanalyst Michael Balint coined the phrase 'the drug doctor' and in both primary and secondary care the physician is the most effective non-pharmacological agent involved in the management of IBS. A patient-centred approach has already been described and emphasized, and this needs to be the first step in management in both settings.

However, informal non-drug therapy continues, with further encounters between IBS patients and their physicians, and the need to 'hold the line' on the diagnosis of IBS is important. Further investigation, referral and reassurance can all become addictive, and a vicious cycle of anxiety, investigation, negative results and further uncertainty can develop, in which everyone concerned – the patient, the doctor and the health-care system – pay a heavy price.

Counselling

> Counselling may be efficacious in IBS patients in whom there is a substantial interplay between social, psychological and physical factors.

Counselling is likely to involve some elements of cognitive therapy, but also focuses on facing and dealing with adverse social and psychological factors. It includes training in relaxation techniques in patients in whom stress is a potent aggravating factor and provides continuing support and explanation for patients confused and worried by their symptoms. Counselling is best undertaken in close collaboration with the patient's primary care physician; many health centres in western Europe now employ counsellors working in parallel with GPs and family physicians.

Counselling is generally undertaken on a one-to-one basis, but this is expensive. Group work for IBS patients may be useful, although there are acknowledged problems in bringing together groups of worried patients with non-organic disorders. Both one-to-one and group-based counselling approaches in primary care have yet to be subjected to randomized controlled trial evaluation.

Cognitive behavioural therapy

Cognitive behavioural therapy (CBT) is a promising technique that is likely to be increasingly applicable in primary care for dealing with a number of non-organic chronic problems. CBT depends on the development of a therapeutic relationship between an individual patient with IBS and a trained cognitive behavioural therapist.

> The cognitive behavioural model for understanding IBS proposes that patients have certain predisposing factors, such as illness beliefs or a reaction to certain foods, that are likely to aggravate IBS.

These symptoms may also be triggered by factors such as stress of concomitant illness; once patients experience further distressing, painful and inconvenient symptoms they may act, think and feel in a way which will maintain and intensify the symptoms. Under conditions of stress IBS patients may have fearful thoughts (cognitions) about the meaning of the symptoms of IBS (Figure 16). This is likely to result in an attempt to control and reduce symptoms which, even if successful in the short term, may lead to reinforcement of fearful thoughts about the uncontrollability or danger of the symptoms. Such patients can become trapped in a vicious cycle of fear and avoidance. Physiological, cognitive and behavioural responses appear to be interdependent and responsible for maintaining the symptoms of the disorder. The cognitive behavioural approach seeks to change patients' cognitions and behaviour in the belief that this will bring about an improvement in the symptoms.

CBT, although used successfully in conditions such as chronic fatigue, is still being evaluated in IBS and results of large randomized controlled trials should be available soon. It seems likely that CBT, particularly when delivered in primary care, will prove to be a useful addition to the range of therapies available.

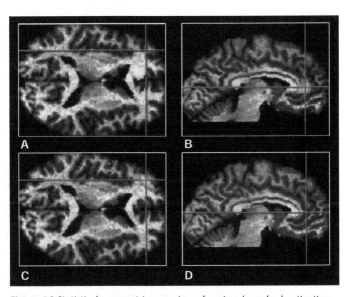

Figure 16 Statistical parametric mapping of regional cerebral activation during anticipation of delivery of painful stimuli. Statistical parametric mapping of pooled activation data from (A and B) all healthy subjects and (C and D) all patients with IBS. Colour-scale corresponds to sites where statistically significant increases in regional activity occurred during (A and C) first and (B and D) second simulated painful stimuli relative to baseline scanning sessions. Modified from Silverman DH et al. *Gastroenterology* 1997;**112**:64–72.

Hypnotherapy

> There is good evidence that so-called gut-directed hypnotherapy is efficacious in the treatment of IBS.

Hypnotherapy has been subjected to randomized controlled trials, but is an expensive option that requires a good deal of training and a number of lengthy sessions of hypnosis. In gut-directed hypnotherapy hypnosis is induced, followed by repeated suggestions of peace and warmth, spreading from a hand on the abdomen, accompanied by the description of relaxing and peaceful mental images, coupled with ego-strengthening suggestions, which are an essential component of hypnotherapy. The IBS patient is also likely to be given audio tapes to take home, so that autohypnosis can be induced at home, to continue treatment after the hypnotherapy sessions have ended.

Complementary therapies

As the response of IBS to traditional drug and non-drug therapies is so erratic, it is not surprising that patients have turned to complementary medical practitioners for help. Complementary approaches include the eradication of *Candida albicans* from the gut using antifungal drugs such as nystatin. Herbal infusions and plant extracts are often used, and their laxative effect may be useful in patients with constipation-predominant IBS. Chinese herbal medicines may be efficacious and a number of other herbal preparations have been recommended for the relief of bloating and flatulence. Pancreatic enzymes have also been recommended in some patients with IBS but are only likely to be effective in patients with genuine pancreatic exocrine insufficiency. There is little literature available to describe or evaluate the impact of other lay or complementary

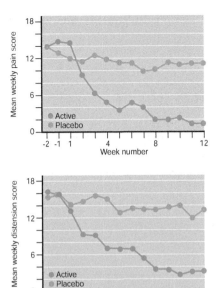

Figure 17 Change in mean weekly scores for abdominal pain in a randomized controlled trial of hypnotherapy. Modified from Whorwell PJ et al. *Lancet* 1984;**2**(8414):1232–4.

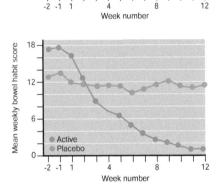

therapists on IBS, although many patients are likely to obtain advice from these sources.

Further reading

Galovski TE, Blanchard EB. The treatment of irritable bowel syndrome with hypnotherapy. *Appl Psychophysiol Biofeedback* 1998;**23**:219–32.

Whorwell PJ, Prior A, Colgan SM. Hypnotherapy in severe irritable bowel syndrome: further experience. *Gut* 1987;**28**:423–5.

Bensoussan A, Talley NJ, Hing M et al. Treatment of irritable bowel syndrome with Chinese herbal medicine: a randomised controlled trial. *JAMA* 1998;**280**:1585–9.

Index

T - #0384 - 101024 - C64 - 187/112/4 - PB - 9781853179853 - Gloss Lamination